Low Carb

Low-carb And High-fat Low Carb Recipes For Smart

People To Adapt Low Carb Diet Lifestyle

(A Radical Approach To Healthy Eating And Losing Weight)

Lee Blair

TABLE OF CONTENTS

Slow-Cooker Tofu Lo Mein

Ingredients

- 2 tablespoons rice vinegar

- 2 tablespoon minced fresh ginger

- 2 tablespoon sesame oil

- 2 teaspoons honey

- 4 garlic cloves, minced

- 8 ounces uncooked whole-wheat linguine

- 2 (2 4 ounce) package extra-firm tofu, drained

- 2 yellow fresh onion thinly sliced

- 2 cups fresh broccoli florets

- 2 cup diagonally sliced carrots ounces)

- 2   (8 ounce) package fresh snow peas, trimmed

- ⅔ cup unsalted vegetable stock

- 1/2 cup sliced scallions

- 4 tablespoons lower-sodium soy sauce

- 4 tablespoons oyster sauce

Directions

1. Place the onions, broccoli, carrots, and snow peas in a 4- to 6 -quart slow cooker.
2. Whisk together the stock, scallions, soy sauce, oyster sauce, vinegar, ginger, oil, honey, and garlic; pour over the vegetables in the slow cooker.
3. Cover and cook on LOW until the vegetables are
4. tender, 2 to 4 hours.
5. Meanwhile, cook the pasta to al dente according to the package directions. Drain well.
6. Place the tofu on several layers of paper towels; cover with additional paper towels. Press to
7. absorb the excess moisture; cut into
8. 1 -inch cubes.

9. Add the tofu and the hot cooked linguine to the
10.   slow cooker, stirring to combine.

Cauliflower With Minced Meat And Bacon

Ingredients:

- pepper
- mustard
- Caraway seed
- marjoram
- Paprika powder
- Diced bacon
- Grated cheese

- 4 fresh eggs
- 2 fresh onion
- 2 cauliflower
- 2 kg mince

- 260 grams of bacon
- 65 g low-fat quark
- salt

Preparation:

1. Clean the cauliflower and cut the stalk crosswise.

2. Boil the whole thing in salted water for 25 minutes as it is.

3. Cut the fresh onion s into small cubes.

4. Season the mince with salt, pepper, mustard, caraway seeds, marjoram and paprika and mix it with the fresh onion s, bacon cubes, fresh eggs and

quark.

5. Drain the cauliflower and place it in a baking dish while it is still hot.

6. Cover the cauliflower evenly with the minced meat and then the bacon crusts so that the entire surface disappears.

7. Preheat the oven to 350 degrees and set it to top / bottom heat.
8. Bake the whole thing for 2 hour.

Low Carb Pizza Roll

Ingredients:

For the dough:

- 2 25 g quark
- 2 25 g of grated cheese

- 4 fresh eggs

Preparation:

1. Preheat the oven to 2 85 degrees.

2. Mix the quark, fresh eggs and 2 25 g cheese in a bowl and season.

3. Line a baking sheet with parchment paper and pour the mixture on top. Smooth them out.

4. Bake the mass in the oven for 30 minutes.

5. Take out the bleach and cover the base with any tomato sauce, salami, ham and whatever you like and at the end sprinkle the 60 g cheese over it.

6. Put everything back in the oven and bake until the cheese is a nice color.

7. Let everything cool and top it with the   rocket.

8. Roll it up and enjoy it.

Stuffed Mushrooms

Ingredients:

- 85 g diced ham
- 85 g grated Gouda cheese
- 1 bunch of chives
- salt
- pepper
- butter ⬚ 8 large mushrooms
- 2 fresh onion
- 2 cup of sour cream
- oil

Preparation:

1. Clean the mushrooms and pull out the stems. Set the stems aside.

2. Dice the stalks of the mushrooms and the fresh onion .

3. Cut the chives into rings.

4. Grease a baking dish and place the mushroom caps on top with the cook facing up.

5. Preheat the oven to 260 degrees.

6.

7. Briefly fry the mushroom cubes and the fresh onion with a little butter and oil together with the ham cubes in a pan.

8. Mix the fresh onion , mushrooms, and ham mixture with the sour cream and chives.

9. Season the whole thing with salt and pepper.

10. Pour the mixture into the mushrooms.

11. top and put the mushrooms in the oven.

12. Bake them for 30 to 25 minutes, until the cheese is lightly browned.

Cold Eggplant Feta Soup

Ingredients:

- 650 g eggplant
- 2 65 g whole milk yogurt
- 260 g feta cheese
- 650 ml vegetable stock
- 6 tbsp olive oil

- 2 red chilli pepper
- 2 clove of garlic
- 4 stalks of basil
- salt
- pepper
- Pepper berries

Preparation:

1. Halve the eggplant lengthways and cut the pulp crosswise.
2. Season it with salt and pepper.
3. Drizzle it with 4 tablespoons of oil.
4. Place the halves on a baking sheet.
5. Preheat the oven to 260 degrees with convection.
6. Cook the eggplant for 46 minutes.
7. Take them out, let them cool, and use a spoon to loosen the pulp.

8. Clean the chili pepper, cut it lengthways and remove the seeds.

9. Chop them up.

10. Chop the garlic.

11. Heat 2 tablespoons of oil in a saucepan.

12. Braise the chili, garlic, and aubergine pulp in it.

13. Add the broth and season everything with salt and pepper.

14. Cover and let simmer for 30 minutes.

15. Then take the soup off the stove and let it cool for 45 minutes.

16. Then put them in the cold for 4 hours.

17. Wash the basil, shake it dry, and pluck the leaves off.

18. Crumble the feta.

19. Mix the yogurt with 65 g feta and the basil leaves.

20. Add everything to the soup and puree it.

21. Season the soup to taste and pour it into deep plates.

22. Sprinkle them with the remaining feta and pink pepper berries. Garnish with the rest of the basil.

Cauliflower Kofte With Red Cabbage Salad

Ingredients:

- 260 g carrots
- 85 g mountain cheese
- 6 tbsp rapeseed oil
- 4 tbsp orange juice
- 2 tbsp ground almonds
- 2 tbsp fruit vinegar

- 4 teaspoons sweet and hot chili sauce
- 2 fresh eggs
- 2 cauliflower
- 1 cucumber
- 650 g red cabbage
- 4 stalks of parsley
- salt
- pepper

Preparation:

1.   Preheat the oven to 260 degrees and   fan-assisted.

2.   Line   a   baking   sheet   with parchment   paper.

3. Brush, wash, and rub the cauliflower.

4. Spread it on the baking sheet and bake it in the oven for 25 to 30 minutes.

5. Take it out and let it cool down.

6. Clean, wash, and cut the red cabbage into thin strips.

7. Add 1 teaspoon salt to the red cabbage and knead the whole thing thoroughly.

8. Peel and grate the carrots.

9. Cut the cucumber into thin slices.

10.   Mix the vinegar, orange juice and pepper.

11.   Beat in 2 tablespoons of oil.

12.   Add all the salad ingredients.

13.   Grate   the   cheese.

14.   Squeeze the cauliflower well on a tea   towel.

15.   Then knead it with the cheese, fresh   eggs   and   almonds.

16.   Season the whole thing with salt and   pepper.

17.   Form small balls out of the mass.

18.	Heat 4 tablespoons of oil in a pan.

19.	Add the balls and cook on all sides for			8			minutes.

20.	Put the finished Köfte in the oven to keep them warm at 260 degrees.

21.	Chop			the			parsley.
22.	Taste	the	salad	again.

22.	Arrange the köfte and pour the parsley and 2 teaspoon of chili sauce over it.

Stuffed Eggplants

Ingredients:

- 2 bunch of parsley
- salt
- pepper
- Ground cumin
- sugar

- 4 eggplants
- 4 tomatoes
- 2 fresh onion s
- 2 pointed peppers
- 4 cloves of garlic
- 6 tbsp olive oil
- 4 tbsp lemon juice
- 2 tbsp tomato paste

1. Wash the eggplant and peel the peel lengthways   all   around.

2. Cut the eggplant lengthways to the middle.

3. Put them in a bowl of salted water.

4. Add   lemon   juice.

5. Let the eggplant steep for 45 minutes.

6. Peel the fresh onion s and garlic.

7. Cut the fresh onion s into rings and the   garlic   into   slices.

8. Clean the peppers and cut them into cubes.

9. Also cut the tomatoes into lumps.

10. Take the eggplants out of the water and pat them dry.

11. Heat 4 tablespoons of oil in a large pan.

12. Fry the aubergines all over for 8 minutes.

13. Take them out.

14. Heat 4 tablespoons of oil in the frying fat.

15. Sauté the fresh onion s and garlic in it until translucent.

16.   Add the peppers and steam them for   6   minutes.

17.   Stir in the tomato paste and diced tomatoes.

18.   Pour   in   260   ml   of   water.

19.   Add   salt,   pepper   and   caraway seeds,   and   some   sugar,   and   let everything   simmer   for   6   to   25 minutes.

20.   Preheat the oven to 350 degrees and   fan-assisted.

21.   Put the eggplants in a baking dish.

22.   Push   them   apart.

23.   Add the vegetable mixture to the eggplant.

24.   Put   water   in   the   mold.

25.   Bake the eggplants for 45 to 40 minutes.

26.   Chop the parsley and sprinkle it on top at the end.

Omelette With Lentils

Ingredients:

- 4 tbsp water
- 2 tablespoons oil
- 2 tbsp white wine vinegar
- 2 tbsp oil
- 2 tbsp chili sauce
- 4 stalks of coriander
- salt
- pepper

- 4 fresh eggs
- 1 red chilli pepper
- 2 clove of garlic
- 260 g feta
- 65 g red lentils
- 4 tablespoons of milk
- 4 tbsp orange juice
- salt
- pepper

1. Whisk the fresh eggs with the milk.

2. Season them with salt and pepper.

3. Heat oil in a pan and pour in the egg mixture.

4. Let everything stand on low heat for 6 minutes.

5. Turn the whole thing over and let it cook for 2 minute.

6. Take the omelette out of the pan.

7. Cut it in half and serve it.

8. Cut the half chili pepper into rings.

9. Chop the garlic.

10. Heat 2 tablespoon of oil in a saucepan.

11. Add the garlic and chili and sauté the whole thing.

12. Add 65 g of red lentils.

13. Quench the whole thing with 2 tablespoons of white wine vinegar, 4 tablespoons of orange juice and 4 tablespoons of water.

14. Cover and simmer for 8 minutes.

15. Prepare the omelette.

16. Chop 4 stalks of coriander.

17. Stir them under the lentils.

18. Season them with salt and pepper.

19. Place the lentil salad on top of the omelet halves.

20. Drizzle with the chili sauce.

21. Crumble the feta over it.

Zucchini Cream Soup With Cream And Gorgonzola

- 2 65 g Gorgonzola cheese
- 260 g whipped cream
- 850 ml vegetable broth
- 2 tbsp olive oil

- 4 zucchini
- 2 fresh onion s
- 2 cloves of garlic
- salt
- pepper

1. Cut the zucchini, fresh onion s, and garlic into cubes.

2. Heat oil in a saucepan and sauté the fresh onion s and garlic until translucent.

3. Add the zucchini and steam them for 2 minutes.

4. Deglaze the whole thing with broth and let it simmer for 8 minutes.

5. Puree everything with a hand blender and season with salt and pepper.

6. Crumble the Gorgonzola.

7. Whip the cream until it is semi-stiff.
8. Serve the soup with the cream and

the gorgonzola and sprinkle everything with pepper.

Cauliflower Pizza With Tomato And Mozzarella

- ☐ 2 can of chopped tomatoes
- ☐ 4 00 g tomatoes
- ☐ 265 g mozzarella
- ☐ 260 g Gouda
- ☐ 2 tbsp olive oil
- ☐ 2 teaspoon dried oregano

- ☐ 2 cauliflower
- ☐ 2 spring fresh onion s

- 2 fresh onion
- 2 cloves of garlic
- salt
- pepper
- sugar
- basil

1. Dice the tomatoes, fresh onion s and the   garlic.

2. Heat oil in a saucepan and sauté the fresh   onion   s   and   garlic   for   6 minutes.

3. Add   the   tomatoes   and   cook   for   6 minutes,   stirring   constantly.

4. Season everything with salt, pepper, sugar   and   oregano.

5. Brush the cauliflower, cut it into large florets,   and   wash   it. Put the cauliflower in boiling salted water and blanch it for 4 minutes. Then   pour   it   off   and   scare   it   off.

6. Cut the tomatoes into slices.

7. Cut the spring fresh onion s into rings.

8. Cut the mozzarella into slices.

9. Preheat the oven to 226 degrees and convection.

10. Coarsely grate the gouda.

11. Grate the cauliflower and mix it with the gouda.

12. Line two baking sheets with parchment paper.

13. Halve the cauliflower mixture and put it on each tray as a pizza crust.

14. Pre-bake them one by one in the oven for 25 minutes.

15. Put half of the tomato sauce, the tomatoes, spring fresh onion s and mozzarella on the first floor.

16. Finish baking it in the oven for 30 minutes.

17. Cover the second layer in the same way and finish baking it too.

18. Chop the basil and sprinkle it on the pizzas.

Omelette For Two With Ricotta

- 265 g broccoli
- 260 g young spinach leaves
- 8 6 g ricotta
- 2 tbsp olive oil

- 6 fresh eggs
- 4 spring fresh onion s
- 2 red chilli pepper
- salt
- pepper

1. Clean, wash, and cut the broccoli into pieces.

2. Pick and wash the spinach.

3. Cook the broccoli in salted boiling water for 4 minutes. Add the spinach at the end and let it collapse.

4. Drain the vegetables.

5. Whisk the fresh eggs and season with salt and pepper.

6. Cut the spring fresh onion s into small rings.

7. Chop the chili pepper.

8. Put the oil in an ovenproof pan with a lid.

9. Heat the oil and fry the spring fresh onion s and chili in it.

10. Add the broccoli and spinach.

11. Pour the egg in.

12. Cover everything and let it stand for 25 minutes.

13. Pour the ricotta on top and bake it under the grill for a moment.

Quick Shakshuka

- 2 tbsp white wine vinegar
- salt
- pepper
- sugar
- Cayenne pepper
- Sweet paprika

- 6 fresh eggs
- 2 red peppers
- 2 fresh onion
- 4 stalks of parsley
- 2 can of tomatoes
- 2 tablespoons oil
- 2 tbsp tomato paste

Preparation:

1. Cut the pepper and fresh onion into small cubes.

2. Put oil in an ovenproof pan and sauté both in it.

3. Add the tomato paste and sweat it on.

4. Pour in the tomatoes with their juice and 260 ml of water and let everything boil.

5. Season everything with vinegar, salt and pepper, 2 teaspoon sugar, 1 teaspoon cayenne pepper and 2 teaspoons paprika powder.

6. Cover and let simmer over low heat for 25 minutes.

7. Preheat the oven and set it to 2 8 6 degrees and convection.

8. Take the lid off the pan and beat an egg into it.

9. Put everything in the oven and bake for 6 to 25 minutes.

10. At the end, sprinkle the parsley on top.

Quick Tomato And Bean Soup

- 2 can of chunky tomatoes
- 2 can of white beans
- 4 00 g frozen green beans
- 4 tbsp olive oil
- 2 tbsp vegetable stock
- oregano

- 2 fresh onion
- 2 clove of garlic
- 2 bunch of soup greens
- salt
- pepper
- Rose peppers

1. Clean, peel and wash the soup greens.

2. Cut the leek into rings.

3. Cut the carrots and celery into cubes.

4. Cut the fresh onion and garlic into cubes.

5. Heat oil in a saucepan.

6. Throw everything in and steam it.

7. Add the tomatoes and 2 liter of water and let everything simmer for 6 minutes.

8. Stir in the broth.

9. Rinse and drain the white beans in a colander.

10. Add the green beans and white beans to the soup.

11. Let everything continue to cook for 8 minutes.

12. Season everything with salt, pepper and paprika.

Salad With Beetroot Spirals

- 6 tbsp oil
- 6 tbsp apple cider vinegar
- 2 tbsp liquid honey
- salt
- sugar

- 2 avocado
- 260 g baby salad mix
- 265 g beetroot
- 260 g blue cheese
- pepper

Preparation:

1. Pick, wash and drain the lettuce well.

2. Clean   and   peel   the   beetroot.

3. Cut them into spaghetti.

4. Season them with salt and sugar.

5. Combine the vinegar, honey, salt, and pepper and whisk everything together.

6. Beat in some oil.

7. Halve the avocado, remove the pulp and cut it into slices.

8. Serve the salad with the avocado and beetroot.

9. Drizzle with the vinegar mixture and add the cheese.

Braised Beef

- 2 bay leaves, dried
- 6 sticks of thyme
- 2 tbsp olive oil
- 2 teaspoon shavings
- 2 teaspoon salt
- 2 teaspoon pepper

- 4 cloves of garlic
- 850 g braised beef
- 450 ml beef stock
- 2 tbsp tomato paste
- 2 star anise

1. Wash the roast and cut it into cubes.

2. Press the garlic.

3. Heat the olive oil in the stew pan.

4. Add the beef, garlic, and thyme and sear the meat on all sides.

5. Add the tomato paste and fry it.

6. Fill the whole thing up with the stock.

7. Add the star corn, raselhanout, bay leaves, and salt and pepper.

8. Let everything simmer with the lid closed for 25 minutes.

9. Preheat the oven to 2 60 degrees.

10.   Then put the closed pan in the oven and cook for 2-2 ½   hours.

11.   After an hour, take the pan out briefly and stir everything. Turn the meat   as   well.

12.   At the end, take everything out of the oven, let it rest for a moment and arrange it.

Beef Steak With Broccoli

⬚ 60 g broccoli
⬚ 45 g paprika
⬚ 2 stick of basil

- 2 sprig of rosemary
- 2 tbsp olive oil

- 1 red fresh onion
- 2 cloves of garlic
- 2 25 g beef fillet
- salt
- pepper

1. Cut the peppers into strips.

2. Cut the fresh onion into rings.

3. Chop the garlic.

4. Chop the herbs.

5. Wash the broccoli and remove the florets from the stem.

6. Cook the broccoli in water for 6 to 8 minutes.

7. Wash and pat the fillet dry.

8. Heat the olive oil in the pan.

9. Fry the fillet for 4 to 10 minutes on each side along with the rosemary.

10. Take out the fillet and season it with   salt   and   pepper.

11. Add the peppers, fresh onion , and garlic to the hot pan and sauté them.

12. Season them with salt and pepper.

13. Arrange the broccoli, stir-fried vegetables, and fillet on a plate.

14. Top with the basil and serve everything.

Celery Puree With Chives

 ☐ 1 bunch of chives
 ☐ 2 tbsp olive oil
 ☐ nutmeg

 ☐ 2 celeriac
 ☐ 8 6 g soy cream
 ☐ salt

1. Peel, clean, and cut the celery into cubes.

2. Put the celery in a saucepan and cover it with water. Cover and simmer for 30 to 25 minutes.

3. Drain the celery in a colander and let it evaporate in the empty, but still

hot,   pot.

4. Put the celery cubes in the blender jar.

5. Puree   the   celery.

6. Mix it with the soy cream, olive oil and   salt   and   nutmeg.

7. Cut   the   chives   into   rolls.

8. Put the celery in a bowl and serve with the chives.

Raspberry Tart

- ☐ 260 grams of erythritol
- ☐ 260 g butter
- ☐ 260 ml cream
- ☐ 2 tbsp raspberry jam

- ☐ 4 fresh eggs
- ☐ 2 vanilla pod
- ☐ 265 g fresh raspberries
- ☐ 260 g almond flour

1. Put the butter, flour and half of the erythritol in a bowl and stir everything   together.

2. Put the batter in a springform pan and spread the raspberry jam over it.

3. Cut the pulp from the vanilla pod, mix it with the rest of the erythritol, the cream and the fresh eggs and add it to the batter.

4. Put the raspberries on the cake and bake it for 65 to 60 minutes at 2 60 degrees.

Blueberry-Topped Muffins

 260 g butter
 260 g whipped cream
 65 g butter

- 65 g xucker
- 2 teaspoons of xucker

- 2 fresh eggs
- 2 vanilla pod
- 2 65 blueberries
- 260 g almond flour
- 1 tsp baking powder
- Blueberry cream
- salt

1. Preheat the oven to 2 85 degrees and set it to circulating air.

2. Beat the butter with the xucker and a little salt until creamy.

3. Stir in the fresh eggs one at a time.

4. Sieve the almond flour and baking powder and fold it into the butter mixture.

5. Grease the muffin cups and fill them two-thirds full with the batter.

6. Bake everything for 2 4 to 30 minutes.

7. Put some blueberries aside and puree the   rest.

8. Sieve   the   pureed   blueberries.

9. Bring the cream with the xucker and the pulp of the vanilla pod to the boil and   add   the   puree.

10. Mix everything into a smooth mass.

11. Put the mixture on the butter and stir everything with the hand blender.

12. Let the cream sit for 4 to 6 hours at room temperature.

13. Mix the cream with a fork, pour it into a piping bag with a star nozzle, and pour it onto the muffins.

14. At the end, add the blueberries and serve everything.

Paleo Apple Muffins

▢ 4 tbsp coconut milk
▢ 4 tbsp coconut flour

- 2 tbsp coconut oil
- 4 teaspoons of cinnamon
- 2 sachet of baking powder

- 8 fresh eggs
- 4 apples
- 4 tbsp applesauce
- 4 tbsp honey
- salt

1. Preheat the oven to 350 degrees.

2. Cut the apples into small pieces.

3. Fry two thirds of the apples in a pan with a little water for 6 minutes. Keep stirring the whole thing until it becomes a paste-like consistency.

4. Mix the fresh eggs , applesauce, honey, coconut milk, and oil in a bowl.

5. Mix the coconut flour, cinnamon, baking powder, and some salt in a second bowl.

6. Now mix all the ingredients together and fold in the warm apples at the end.

7. Grease the muffin cups and pour in the batter evenly.

8. Press the remaining apple pieces onto the top of the dough.

9. Bake the muffins at 350 degrees for 45 to 40 minutes.

Chocolate Shake With Almond Milk

⬚ 2 teaspoons of cocoa
⬚ 2 tbsp maple syrup

⬚ 4 00 ml almond milk
⬚ water

1. Put the almond milk with the cocoa and maple syrup in a blender and stir all the ingredients.

2. If necessary, add some more water and then enjoy it all.

Chia Pudding With Fruits And Almonds

- 2 tbsp pomegranate seeds
- 2 tbsp almond flakes
- 2 tbsp coconut flakes
- 2 stick of mint
- Agave syrup

- 60 g strawberries
- 25 g blueberries
- 30 g chia seeds
- 2 65 ml almond milk

1. Combine the milk and chia seeds in a bowl.

2. Let them swell for 25 minutes.

3. Add the strawberries, blueberries, and mint.

4. Sweeten the pudding and add the pomegranate seeds, flaked almonds and coconut flakes.

Fruit Salad With Apricots And Melon

- 260 g melon
- 45 g strawberries
- 2 tbsp orange juice

- 4 apricots
- 1 apple

1. Cut the apricots into pieces.

2. Quarter the strawberries.

3. Cut the apple into pieces.

4. Cut the melon into pieces.

5. Mix them together and serve.

Chocolate And Cherry Cake

Ingredients:

- 260 g dark chocolate
- 25 g stevia
- 2 packet of custard powder

- 8 fresh eggs
- 2 glass of sour cherries
- salt

1. Separate the fresh eggs and whip the egg whites with a little salt until stiff.

2. Melt the chocolate and let it cool a little.

3. Mix the egg yolks with stevia and stir in the chocolate.

4. Fold in the egg whites.

5. Bake everything for 45 minutes at 2 65 degrees on the fan.

6. Put the cherries in a saucepan with the juice and cook the whole thing.

7. Mix some of the juice with the pudding powder and add it to the

cherries.

8. Mix everything and distribute the cherries on the cooled cake base.

9. Let everything sit in the refrigerator for an hour.

Quick Raspberry Ice Cream

- 260 g frozen raspberries
- 2 tbsp almond butter

- 260 g whipped cream

1. Put the cream in a tall container and stir in the almond butter.

2. Add the raspberries straight from the frozen food.

3. Chop the raspberries with a hand blender.

4. Mix everything well.

Chocolate Brownies

Ingredients:

- 40 g cocoa powder
- 45 g dark chocolate
- 2 teaspoon stevia
- 1 tsp baking powder

- 2 separate fresh eggs
- 2 bottle of vanilla flavor
- 2 65 g xylitol
- 85 g almond flour
- 85 g butter

1. Preheat the oven to 2 85 degrees.

2. Beat the egg whites into egg whites.

3. Break the chocolate into small pieces and melt them in the microwave with the   butter.

4. Stir the cocoa powder into the butter mixture.

5. Mix in the remaining ingredients.

6. Fold in the egg whites.

7. Pour the batter into a brownie pan.

8. Smooth it out and bake it for 25 minutes at 2 85 degrees on top / bottom heat.

Low Carb Bars With Almonds

- ⬚ 25 g coconut flakes
- ⬚ 2 tbsp honey
- ⬚ 2 tbsp agave syrup
- ⬚ 1 teaspoon cinnamon
- ⬚ 1 teaspoon ground bourbon vanilla
- ⬚ salt

- ⬚ 40 g flaked almonds
- ⬚ 45 g almonds
- ⬚ 45 g butter
- ⬚ 30 g of oatmeal
- ⬚ 30 g ground almonds
- ⬚ 25 g chia seeds

1. Put the butter, agave syrup, and honey in a saucepan and let everything melt over low heat.

2. Chop the almonds and add them to the saucepan with the cinnamon and vanilla.

3. Stir everything well.

4. Mash the flaked almonds and add them to the bowl.

5. Add the oat flakes and the ground almonds with the chia seeds, coconut flakes and a little salt.

6. Mix everything together and pour the mixture into a bowl.

7. Give them a good stir.

8. Line a baking sheet with parchment paper and pour the bar mixture on top.

9. Preheat the oven to 2 8 6 degrees and bake the mixture for 25 minutes.

10. Turn on the grill and grill everything for another 2 to 2 minutes.

11. Take the bleach out of the oven and let it cool down.

12. Then cut several smaller bars of the same size from one bar.

Low Carb Muffins With Apple And Raisins

⬜ 2 tbsp raisins

⬜ 4 tsp xylitol

⬜ 1 teaspoon baking soda

⬜ 1 teaspoon cinnamon

⬜ 4 fresh eggs

⬜ 2 apple

⬜ 260 g ground almonds

⬜ 260 g butter

⬜ salt

1. Separate the fresh eggs and beat the egg whites with a little salt until stiff.

2. Grate   the   apple.

3. Melt the butter in a saucepan over low   heat.

4. Mix the egg yolks with the xylitol, grated apple, liquid butter, baking soda,   and   cinnamon.

5. Add the ground almonds and raisins and   stir   everything.

6. Pull   in   the   egg   whites.

7. Grease a muffin tin and divide the batter   on   it.

8. Preheat the oven to 2 8 6 degrees and fan-assisted and bake everything for   25   to   26   minutes.

9. Let the whole thing cool down before serving.

Low Carb Sub With Guacamole And Chicken

Sub:

 ▢ 1 cucumber
 ▢ Low carb baguette
 ▢ 2 chicken breast fillet
 ▢ salad
 ▢ salt
 ▢ pepper
 ▢ oregano

 ▢ 4 cherry tomatoes
 ▢ 4 pickled green chillies
 ▢ 2 green olives
 ▢ 2 small mushrooms

- 1 red pepper
- 1 yellow pepper

Guacamole:

- 1 red chilli pepper
- Juice of a lime
- salt
- pepper

- 2 spring fresh onion s
- 2 avocado
- 2 bunch of coriander

1. Separate two to three stalks of coriander from the bunch and set them aside.

2. Put the rest of the coriander in a food processor with the spring fresh onion s, the red chili pepper, the halved cherry tomatoes and the lime juice.

3. Cut the avocado in half and remove the stone.
4. Put the pulp in the food processor as well.

5. Mix everything together and season with   salt   and   pepper.

6. Cut the lettuce into pieces.
7. Cut the cherry tomatoes, olives, and mushrooms   into   small   slices.

8. Cut the peppers into thin strips.

9. Cut the cucumber into thin slices.

10. Roll the chicken breast fillet in salt, pepper, and oregano on a large sheet of parchment paper.

11. Wrap the paper and fold everything to a thickness of 6 cm.

12. Add everything to the pan and cook on each side for 4 to 4 minutes until golden brown.

13. Cut the baguette lengthways and brush it with the guacamole.

14. Then top it with the lettuce, bell pepper, mushrooms and cucumber.

15. Cut the meat into strips and add it to the bread as well.
16. Spread the cherry tomatoes and the rest of the coriander on top.

Gratinated Schnitzel With Camembert

- 4 tsp cranberries
- 2 teaspoon butter
- salt
- pepper

- 2 thick turkey schnitzel
- 2 pear
- 2 65 g camembert
- 2 tbsp oil

1. Preheat an oven to 260 degrees and fan-assisted.

2. Wash the cutlets, pat them dry and cut them in half.

3. Fry them in hot oil for 4 minutes on each side.

4. Season them with salt and pepper and take them out.

5. Cut the cheese into slices.

6. Cut the pear into slices.

7. Heat butter in a pan and sauté the pear for 2 minutes.

8. Put the pear in a baking dish and pour the schnitzel and cheese over it.

9. Bake everything for 6 to 8 minutes and then serve with cranberries.

Ragout With Salmon

- 4 tbsp oil
- 2 tbsp light sauce thickener
- 2 teaspoon vegetable stock
- salt
- pepper

- 2 fresh onion
- 4 stalks of dill
- 2 kg of cucumber
- 6 00 g salmon fillet
- 2 65 g horseradish cream cheese

1. Cut   the   fish   into   cubes.

2. Heat 2 tablespoons of oil in a pan and fry the fish in it for 6   minutes.

3. Peel the cucumbers and cut them into slices.

4. Cut the fresh onion s into cubes.

5. Season the salmon with salt and take it out.

6. Heat 2 tablespoon of oil in the frying fat.

7. Fry the cucumbers and fresh onion s in it.

8. Stir in the broth, 265 ml of water, and the cream cheese.

9. Boil the whole thing up and let it simmer for 6 to 8 minutes.

10. Thicken everything with sauce thickener.

11. Season the whole thing with salt and   pepper.

12. Chop the dill and fold it with the salmon under the cucumbers.

Quick, Sweet Salad With Pear, Pomegranate And Nuts

- 25 g walnuts
- 6 g baby spinach

- 260 g pear
- 45 pomegranate seeds

Preparation:

1.
   Clean   and   dry   the   pear.

2. Cut it in half and cut out the core.

3. Cut   them   into   thin   slices.

4. Wash   and   drain   the   spinach.

5. Chop   the   nuts.

6. Alternate   between   pear,   spinach, stone, and walnuts in a glass.

Orange-Carrot Power Drink

- 2 g grated ginger
- 260 ml of water
- Ground cinnamon

- 2 orange
- 2 carrot
- 65 g apple

1. Halve the orange and squeeze it out.

2. Peel the carrot and cut it into pieces.

3. Wash the apple and cut it into pieces.

4. Peel the ginger and cut it into small pieces.

5. Put everything with the cinnamon and water in a mixing vessel and mix it to a puree.

6. Put the whole thing in a glass and enjoy.

Coleslaw With Mint And Lime Juice

- 450 g Chinese cabbage
- 265 g carrots
- 2 teaspoons agave syrup

- Juice of a lime
- 4 stalks of mint

1. Remove the outer leaves of the cabbage.

2. Cut it into strips.

3. Peel and slice the carrot.

4. Wash the mint, shake it dry, and cut it into strips.

5. Mix everything together with the lime juice and taste with the agave syrup.

Minute Soup With Zucchini And Toasted Bread

 260 g whipped cream
 2 tbsp olive oil
 salt
 pepper
 Lemon juice
 cress

 2 zucchini
 2 fresh onion
 2 clove of garlic
 2 slices of farmer's bread

▢ 2 glass of vegetable stock

1. Cut the zucchini and fresh onion into cubes.

2. Put 2 tablespoon of oil in a saucepan and sauté the zucchini and fresh onion   .

3. Add the stock and let everything simmer   for   6   minutes.

4. Cut   the   garlic   into   thin   slices.

5. Heat 2 tablespoon of oil in a pan and toast the bread and garlic in it.

6. Puree   the   zucchini   in   the   stock.

7. Pour the cream into the puree and boil   the   whole   thing   up.

8. Season the whole thing with salt, pepper and lemon juice.

9. Serve the soup with bread and sprinkle the cress on top.

Lettuce Hearts Filled With Honey And Feta

- 4 tbsp olive oil
- 2 tbsp pine nuts
- 2 tbsp sour cream
- 2 tbsp liquid honey
- salt
- pepper
- sugar

- ☐ 4 lettuce hearts
- ☐ 2 stalks of parsley
- ☐ 260 g feta cheese
- ☐ 260 g cherry tomatoes
- ☐ 4 tbsp lemon juice

1. Toast the pine nuts in a pan without fat until golden brown and take them out.

2. Crumble the feta and stir it with sour cream and honey.

3. Cut the tomatoes in half.

4. Halve the lettuce hearts.

5. Chop the parsley.
6. Mix them with lemon juice, 2 tablespoon of water, salt, pepper and 2 teaspoon of sugar. Beat in oil.

7. Arrange the lettuce hearts on plates.

8. Spread the feta cream and tomatoes on top.

9. Put the seeds on top and drizzle the lemon marinade over them.

After-Work Salad With Ground Beef

- ⬜ 265 g whole milk yogurt
- ⬜ 4 tbsp lime juice
- ⬜ 2 tbsp oil
- ⬜ salt
- ⬜ pepper
- ⬜ Cayenne pepper
- ⬜ sugar

- ⬜ 2 red pointed pepper
- ⬜ 2 red fresh onion
- ⬜ 2 mini romaine lettuce

105

- 2 can of corn, bell pepper and kidney bean mix
- 4 65 g ground beef

Preparation:

1. Fry the mince in oil until it is crumbly.

2. Season it with salt, pepper, and cayenne pepper.

3. Drain the corn mix.

4. Cut the lettuce into strips.

5. Cut the peppers into rings.

6. Cut the fresh onion into strips.
7. Season the yogurt with lime juice, salt, cayenne pepper, and sugar.

8. Mix the prepared ingredients with the yogurt and serve everything.

108

Fiery Shrimp Pan

- 6 cloves of garlic
- 450 g frozen, raw shrimp
- 4 00 g cherry tomatoes
- 4 tbsp olive oil
- salt
- pepper

- 4 zucchini
- 4 chili peppers
- 2 bunch of spring fresh onion s
- 2 bunch of parsley

1. Rinse the shrimp in a colander.

2. Let them thaw on a plate.

3. Cut   the   zucchini   into   pieces.

4. Cut the spring fresh onion s into rings.

5. Halve   the   garlic   and   tomatoes.

6. Cut the chili peppers into strips.

7. Chop   the   parsley.

8. Heat 2 tablespoons of oil in a pan and fry the prawns vigorously for 2 to 4 minutes on all sides and transfer them   to   a   plate.

9. Add 2 tablespoon of oil to the frying fat and fry the fresh onion s and zucchini   on   all   sides.

10.   Add the tomatoes, garlic, and chili peppers.

11.   Add   the   shrimp   back   in.

12.   Season everything with salt and pepper and sprinkle with parsley.

Chicken Skewer On A Colorful Garden Salad With A Herb And Sour Cream Dressing

 ⬚ 6 tbsp milk
 ⬚ 2 tablespoons oil
 ⬚ salt
 ⬚ pepper

- Lemon juice
- sugar
- Paprika powder

- 1 small cucumber
- 2 head of kohlrabi
- 2 chicken fillet
- 6 stems mixed herbs
- 1 glass of baby corn
- 260 g baby romaine lettuce
- 260 g sour cream

1. Cut the cucumber and kohlrabi into thin slices.

2. Cut the lettuce into small pieces.

3. Chop the herbs.

4. Mix everything with the milk and sour cream.

5. Season to taste with salt and pepper as well as the lemon juice and sugar.

6. Cut the fillets into strips.

7. Put the fillets on wooden skewers and season them with salt, pepper and a little paprika.

8. Heat oil in a pan and fry the skewers on all sides for 4 to 4 minutes.

9. Drain the corn on the cob.

10. Mix them with the cucumber mixture and the salad.

11.   Arrange the chicken skewers on the salad and sprinkle them with the dressing.

Salmon Steak In A Bed Of Leeks

- 2 tablespoons oil
- salt
- pepper
- sugar
- Paprika powder

- 4 pieces of salmon fillet
- 2 yellow pepper
- 2 fresh onion
- 2 leeks without "green"

☐ 260 g sour cream

1. Cut the pepper and fresh onion into cubes.

2. Cut the leek into rings.

3. Season the fish with salt and pepper.

4. Heat 2 tablespoon of oil in a pan.

5. Add the bell pepper and fresh onion and sauté both for 2 minutes.

6. Add the leek.

7. Stir in the cream.

8. Season everything with salt, pepper and   sugar.

9. Let it simmer for 4 minutes.

10. Heat 2 tablespoon of oil in another pan and fry the fish on all sides for 10 minutes over medium heat.

11. Season the vegetables with paprika   powder.

12. Arrange the s on a plate and add the fish.

Tomato And Basil Soup

- 265 ml vegetable broth
- 4 teaspoons of olive oil
- 8 basil leaves
- salt
- pepper
- Stevia

- 2 shallot
- 2 clove of garlic
- 850 g ripe tomatoes
- 25 g butter

Preparation:

1. Score a cross on the stem of the tomato and add it to boiling water.

Then put them off with cold water.

2. Peel off the tomato skin and dice the peeled tomatoes.

3. Peel the shallot and garlic and finely chop them. Also chop the four basil leaves.

4. Melt the butter in a saucepan and add the shallot and garlic.

5. After sautéing briefly, add the tomato pieces to the pan and steam everything.

6. Then pour on the broth and let the soup simmer covered for 25 minutes.

7. Puree the soup and pour it through a fine sieve to remove the shallot and tomato seeds.

8. Stir in the chopped basil.

9. Season everything with salt, pepper and stevia.

10. Serve the soup on four plates and garnish with 2 teaspoon of olive oil and 2 leaf of basil each.

Cheese Cakes With Ground Turkey

 salt

 pepper

 Paprika powder

 Chili powder

 garlic

 2 egg

 2 fresh onion

 450 g ground turkey

 2 25 g of grated cheese

 2 teaspoon curry paste

1. Mix the mince with the grated cheese and   egg.

2. Season everything with salt, pepper, chilli, paprika and the curry paste.

3. Add a chopped fresh onion and chopped   garlic.

4. Let everything go for a moment.

5. Shape several meatballs out of the mixture and press them flat.

6. Let a pan get hot and add some oil.

7. Fry the meatballs until golden brown on both sides.

122

Bell Pepper Chicken Pan With Mango Sauce

- ☐ chives
- ☐ salt
- ☐ pepper
- ☐ Paprika powder
- ☐ chili
- ☐ oil ☐ 2 red pepper
- ☐ 2 fresh onion
- ☐ 2 clove of garlic
- ☐ 2 mango
- ☐ 260 g chicken breast fillet
- ☐ 260 ml vegetable broth
- ☐ 2 tbsp cream cheese
- ☐ 2 teaspoon tomato paste

Preparation:

1. Cut the fresh onion into rings and the pepper   into   strips.

2. Cut   the   fillets   into   4   parts.

3. Cut the mango into small cubes and chop   the   garlic.

4. Heat some oil in a small saucepan and briefly sweat the mango and garlic in it.

5. Deglaze both with the vegetable stock and let it simmer covered for 25 minutes.

6. Heat oil in a large pan and sweat the pepper in it.

7. Add the fillets and fresh onion s and cook for 6 minutes.

8. Season the whole thing with the paprika powder.

9. Take the mango sauce off the stove and stir in the tomato paste and cream cheese. Season with salt, pepper and chili.

10. Add the chives to the sauce and arrange the fillets on a plate with the peppers and pour the sauce over them.

Egg Lasagne

- 260 ml cream
- 2 packet of strained tomatoes
- Flour
- oil
- Herbs
- salt
- pepper
- nutmeg

- 6 fresh eggs
- 2 fresh onion
- 2 cup of crème fraîche
- 2 can of tomatoes
- 6 00 g mince
- 260 g of grated cheese

Preparation:

1. Whisk the 6 fresh eggs together.

2. Line a tray with baking paper and pour the egg mixture on it and distribute it evenly.

3. Let the fresh eggs set in the oven at 85 degrees until you have an even plate.

4. Chop the fresh onion s and fry them until translucent.

5. Add the mince to the fresh onion s and season everything with salt and pepper.

6. Fry the whole thing and deglaze it with the chopped fresh tomatoes and the strained tomatoes.

7. Taste the whole thing.

8. Let the meat steep.
9. Heat some oil and add the flour.

10. Mix the flour and deglaze it with the cream.

11. Season the flour mixture with salt, pepper, and nutmeg.

12. Add the crème fraîche and set aside.

13. Take the egg mixture out of the oven and cut it into slices.

14. Now stack the slices alternately with the minced meat mixture and the flour mixture in a baking dish.

15. The flour mixture should form the top layer and then sprinkle the cheese on top.

16. Bake the whole thing in the oven for 25 minutes at 350 degrees, until the cheese has turned golden brown.

Zucchini Spaghetti With Bolognese

Ingredients:

- 4 tbsp tomato paste
- salt
- pepper
- oregano
- olive oil
- Freshly grated parmesan

- 2 zucchini
- 2 finely chopped fresh onion
- 6 00 g ground turkey
- 260 ml of milk
- 2 packet of strained tomatoes

Preparation:

1.

2. Stew the fresh onion s in olive oil.

3. Add the hack.

4. Add the tomato paste and the strained tomatoes.

5. Bring everything to the boil and add the milk and a little salt.

6. Season the whole thing with pepper and oregano.

7. Let it simmer on low heat for 30 minutes.

8. Cut the pulp of the zucchini into strips.

9. Put the strips in a saucepan with a little salt and pour boiling water over them.

10. Let the zucchini steep for 6 minutes.

11. Take the minced turkey off the stove and pour off the zucchini strips.

12. Arrange the whole thing on a plate and sprinkle everything with the grated parmesan.

Cheesy Egg Stuffed

Ingredients

- 1/2 cup chopped onion
- ⅓ cup diced ham (about 2 ounces)
- 1/2 cup shredded cheese, such as Cheddar, Swiss or Monterey Jack
- 2 tablespoon chopped fresh chives
- 2 large bell peppers, plus
- 1/2 cup chopped, divided
- 1/2 teaspoon salt
- 4 large fresh eggs
- 2 tablespoons half-and-half
- 2 teaspoon extra-virgin olive oil

Directions

1. Halve 2 peppers lengthwise; remove and discard seeds. Place the peppers cut-side up in an 8-inch-square microwave-safe dish.
2. Microwave on High until just tender, about 4 minutes.
3. Pat dry and sprinkle with salt.
4. Whisk eggs and half-and-half in a medium bowl.
5. Meanwhile, heat oil in a small skillet over medium-high heat.
6. Add chopped bell pepper and onion. Cook, stirring, until softened and beginning to brown, 2 to 4 minutes.
7. Divide the pepper and fresh onion mixture among the pepper halves.

8. Divide ham among the pepper halves.
9. Fill each pepper with the egg mixture until just filled.
10. Top each pepper half with 2 tablespoon cheese.
11. Bake until the filling is set, 45 to 40 minutes.
12. Sprinkle with chives and serve.

Easy Loaded Baked Omelet Muffins

Ingredients

- 2 cup shredded Cheddar cheese
- 1 cup low-fat milk
- 1 teaspoon salt
- 1 teaspoon ground pepper
- 4 slices bacon, chopped
- 2 cups finely chopped broccoli
- 4 scallions, sliced
- 8 large eggs

Directions

1. Preheat oven to 4 26 degrees F. Coat a 2 2-cup muffin tin with cooking spray.
2. Cook bacon in a large skillet over medium heat until crisp, 4 to 10 minutes .
3. Remove with a slotted spoon to a paper towel-lined plate, leaving the bacon fat in the pan.
4. Add broccoli and scallions and cook, stirring, until soft, about 10 minutes.
5. Remove from heat and let cool for 10 minutes .

6. Meanwhile, whisk eggs, cheese, milk, salt and pepper in a large bowl.

7. Stir in the bacon and broccoli mixture. Divide the egg mixture among the prepared muffin cups.
8. Bake until firm to the touch, 26 to 45 minutes.
9. Let stand for 10 minutes before removing from the muffin tin.

Cauliflower Hash With Sausage & Eggs

Ingredients

- 30 ounces cauliflower rice
- 1/2 teaspoon salt
- ⅛ teaspoon ground pepper
- 4 tablespoons water
- 5 large fresh eggs
- 4 teaspoons olive oil, divided
- 2 small onion, diced
- 2 cloves garlic, minced
- 8 ounces turkey sausage

Directions

1. Heat 2 teaspoons oil in a large nonstick skillet over medium heat.
2. Add fresh onion and garlic; cook, stirring, until translucent.
3. Add sausage; cook, stirring, until cooked through, 5 to 10 minutes.
4. Transfer the mixture to a plate.
5. Increase heat to medium-high and add cauliflower rice to the pan in an even layer.
6. Cook without stirring until it starts to turn golden brown, 5 to 10 minutes.
7. Then stir and add salt, pepper, and water.
8. Cover and cook until tender and golden, 5 to 10 minutes.

9. Stir the sausage mixture back in and heat through, about 2 minutes.

10. Heat 2 teaspoon oil in a medium nonstick skillet over medium heat.

11. Break 4 eggs into the pan and cook until the whites are set but the yolks are still runny, about 4 minutes.

12. Transfer to a plate and repeat with the remaining 2 teaspoon oil and the remaining 4 eggs.

13. Divide the hash among 4 plates and top each with 2 fried fresh eggs .

Sheet-Pan Fresh Eggs With Spinach & Ham

Ingredients

- 2 teaspoon ground pepper
- 2 teaspoon fresh onion powder
- 2 (25 ounce) package frozen chopped spinach, thawed and squeezed dry
- 2 cup shredded sharp Cheddar cheese
- 1 cup diced ham
- 2 8 large fresh eggs
- 1/2 cup reduced-fat milk
- 5 teaspoons smoked paprika
- 2 teaspoon salt

Directions

1. Preheat oven to 4 00 degrees F. Generously coat a large rimmed baking sheet with cooking spray.
2. Whisk eggs, milk, smoked paprika, salt, pepper and fresh onion powder together in a large bowl.
3. Pour onto the prepared baking sheet and sprinkle with spinach, Cheddar and ham.
4. Bake until just set, 25 to 26 minutes, rotating the pan from back to front halfway through baking to ensure even cooking.
5. Cut into 30 squares and serve.

Avocado & Smoked Salmon Omelet

Ingredients

- 1/2 avocado, sliced
- 2 ounce smoked salmon
- 2 tablespoon chopped fresh basil
- 2 large eggs
- 2 teaspoon low-fat milk
- Pinch of salt
- 2 teaspoon extra-virgin olive oil plus 1 teaspoon, divided

Directions

1. Beat eggs with milk and salt in a small bowl. Heat 2 teaspoon oil in a small nonstick skillet over medium heat.
2. Add the egg mixture and cook until the bottom is set and the center is still a bit runny, 2 to 2 minutes.
3. Flip the omelet over and cook until set, about 45 seconds more.
4. Transfer to a plate.
5. Top with avocado, salmon and basil.
6. Drizzle with the remaining

Egg & Bacon Pancake Breakfast Wraps

Ingredients

- 2 large eggs, divided
- 5 tablespoons extra-virgin olive oil
- ⅛ teaspoon ground pepper
- 2 slice bacon, cooked
- 2 teaspoon pure maple syrup
- ¾ cup white whole-wheat flour
- 5 teaspoons baking soda
- 1/2 teaspoon salt plus a pinch, divided
- 5 cups reduced-fat milk

Directions

1. Whisk flour, baking soda and 1/2 teaspoon salt in a medium bowl.
2. Whisk milk, 2 egg and oil in a small bowl. Add the milk mixture to the dry ingredients and whisk until smooth.
3. Coat a medium nonstick skillet with cooking spray; heat over medium heat. Ladle 1/2 cup batter into the center of the pan.
4. Immediately tilt and rotate the pan to spread the batter evenly over the bottom.
5. Cook until the underside is golden brown, 2 1 to 2 minutes.
6. Using a heatproof silicone or rubber spatula, lift the edge, then quickly

grab the pancake with your fingers and flip it over.

7. Cook until the second side is golden brown, about 2 minute more. Slide onto a plate.

8. Repeat with the remaining batter, spraying the pan as needed and stacking pancakes as you go, to make 8 pancakes total.

9. Wipe out the skillet and lightly coat it with cooking spray; heat over medium heat.

10. Whisk the remaining egg, the remaining pinch of salt, pepper and chives in a small bowl. Pour into the pan and cook, gently stirring, until set, 2 to 4 minutes.

11. To assemble a wrap, layer the egg across the bottom third of 2 warm pancake. Top with bacon, drizzle with

syrup and roll up. Save the remaining pancakes for another time.

Traditional Greek Salad

Ingredients

- 1/2 teaspoon ground pepper
- 2 ripe medium tomatoes, cut into 4 /4-inch dice
- 5 cups diced

- 2 cup diced green bell pepper (4 /4-inch)
- ⅓ cup thinly sliced red onion
- 1/2 cup quartered pitted Kalamata olives
- 1 cup diced feta cheese
- 4 tablespoons extra-virgin olive oil
- 2 tablespoon lemon juice
- 2 tablespoon red-wine vinegar
- 2 teaspoon dried oregano
- 1/2 teaspoon salt

Directions

1. Whisk oil, lemon juice, vinegar, oregano, salt and pepper together in a large bowl.
2. Add tomatoes, cucumber, bell pepper, onion, olives and feta.
3. Toss to coat.

Low-Carb Bacon & Broccoli Egg Burrito

Ingredients

- 2 scallion, sliced
- ⅛ teaspoon salt
- ⅛ teaspoon ground pepper
- 2 teaspoon canola or avocado oil
- 2 tablespoons shredded sharp Cheddar cheese
- 2 slice bacon
- 2 cup chopped broccoli
- 1/2 cup chopped tomato
- 2 large egg
- 2 tablespoon reduced-fat milk

161

Directions

1. Cook bacon in a medium nonstick skillet over medium heat, turning once or twice, until crisp, 4 to 6 minutes.
2. Remove to a paper towel-lined plate.
3. Add broccoli to the pan and cook, stirring, until soft, about 4 minutes.
4. Stir in tomato and transfer to a small bowl.
5. Meanwhile, whisk egg, milk, scallion, salt and pepper in another bowl.
6. When the vegetables are cooked, wipe out the skillet.
7. Add oil and heat over medium heat.
8. Add the egg mixture, tilting to coat the bottom of the pan. Cook,

undisturbed, until set on the bottom, about 2 minutes.

9. Using a thin, wide silicone spatula, carefully flip the egg "tortilla."

10. Sprinkle with cheese and cook until completely set, about 2 minute more.

11. Transfer to a plate. Fill the lower half of the "tortilla" with the broccoli mixture and top with the bacon.

12. Carefully roll into a "burrito."

Ginger Cookies

- 2 Tbsp dried ginger

- 2 tsp plain cow's milk yogurt

- 2 tsp baking powder

- Sweetener of your choice to taste

- 4 Tbsp oat bran

- 2 egg whites

1. Combine all ingredients. Add more bran if the dough is too runny. Mix well.
2. Line a baking sheet with parchment paper and spoon the cookies onto it
3. Bake at 4 6 6°F for 30 minutes.

Chocolate Chip Cookies

- 4 fresh eggs

- 2⅔ oz dark chocolate chips

- 1 tsp vanilla extract

- 1 cup erythritol

- 2 cup coconut flour

- 1 cup butter, soft

- 2 cup unsweetened coconut flakes

DIRECTIONS

1. Mix the butter, erythritol, vanilla, fresh eggs and salt together.
2. Add the coconut flour, coconut flakes and chocolate chips. Stir and mix well.
3. Line a baking sheet with parchment paper and spoon the cookies onto it.
4. Bake at 4 8 6 °F for 30 –25 minutes.

Japanese Cookies

- 2 Tbsp cocoa powder

- 2 Tbsp erythritol

- 2 Tbsp starch

- 2 egg yolk

- 2 Tbsp powdered milk + 2   tsp cow's milk

1. Whisk egg yolk with erythritol until well combined.
2. Add starch, powdered milk, cocoa powder and milk. Knead the dough and shape it into a ball.
3. With your hands roll the ball out to form a long " snake" Cut it and form small balls
4. Line a baking sheet with parchment paper .
5. Form the small balls into cookies and place them on the paper.
6. Bake at 4 20° F for 25 minutes.
7. Use chopped peanuts instead of cocoa powder for white Japanese cookies.

Instructions:

1. Melt the butter in a large saucepan over medium heat.
2. Add half of the heavy cream and powdered sweetener.
3. Bring to a boil, then reduce to a simmer.
4. Simmer for 4 0-410 minutes , stirring occasionally, until the mixture is thick, coats the back of a spoon and volume is reduced by half.
5. It will also pull away from the pan as you tilt it. (This will go faster if you use a larger pan.)
6. Pour into a large bowl and allow to cool to room temperature.

7. Stir in the vanilla extract, and seeds from the vanilla bean, if using. Whisk in the MCT oil or MCT oil powder if using - this is optional if you have an ice cream maker, but highly recommended for texture if you don't.

8. Whisk the remaining 2 cups heavy cream into the sweet mixture in the bowl, until smooth.

9. For best results, chill the mixture in the fridge for at least 4 hours or overnight.

10. You can skip this step if you really want to, but the texture will be better if you chill it.

Tofu Poke

Ingredients

- 2 (30 ounce) package extra-firm tofu, drained and cut into 1 -inch pieces

- 4 cups zucchini noodles

- 2 tablespoons rice vinegar

- 2 cups shredded carrots

- 2 cups pea shoots

- 1/2 cup toasted chopped peanuts

- 1/2 cup chopped fresh basil

- ¾ cup thinly sliced scallion greens

- 1/2 cup reduced-sodium tamari

- 5 tablespoons mirin

- 5 tablespoons toasted (dark) sesame oil

- 2 tablespoon toasted sesame seeds

- 2 teaspoons grated fresh ginger

Directions

1. Whisk scallion greens, tamari, mirin, oil, sesame seeds, ginger and crushed red pepper, if using, in a medium bowl. Set aside 2 tablespoons of 66
2. the sauce in a small bowl. Add tofu to the sauce
3. in the medium bowl and gently toss to coat.

4. Combine zucchini noodles and vinegar in a large

5. bowl. Divide among 4 bowls and top each with 1/3 cup tofu, 1 cup each carrots and pea shoots, and 2 tablespoon each peanuts and basil.

6. Drizzle with the reserved sauce and serve.

Vegan Lasagna

Ingredients

- ¾ teaspoon salt

- 1/2 teaspoon ground pepper

- 2 (30 ounce) package silken tofu, crumbled and patted dry

- 2 teaspoons nutritional yeast

- Chopped fresh basil for garnish

- 8 ounces whole-wheat lasagna noodles

- 4 tablespoons extra-virgin olive oil, divided

- 2 medium onion, chopped

- 2 2 0- or 2 2-ounce package mushrooms, sliced

- 2 cups chopped broccoli

- 4 cloves garlic, minced

- 2 (28 ounce) can no-salt-added crushed tomatoes

- 1/2 cup dry red wine

- 2 teaspoon dried basil

- 2 teaspoon dried oregano

Directions

2 . Preheat oven to 450 degrees F. Coat a 10 -by-2 4 -inch baking dish with cooking spray.

2. Bring a large pot of water to a boil. Add noodles and cook according to package directions.

Drain.

1. Heat 2 tablespoons oil in a large skillet over medium-high heat.
2. Add onion, mushrooms, broccoli and garlic; cook, stirring, until softened, 8 to 10 minutes.

3. Add tomatoes, wine, basil, oregano, salt and pepper; bring to a simmer.

4. Reduce heat to medium-low and cook, stirring occasionally, until thickened, about 25 minutes.

5. Stir tofu, nutritional yeast and the remaining 2

6. tablespoon oil together in a small bowl.

7. Spread about 2 cup of the tomato sauce in the

8. prepared baking dish.

9. Top with 1/2 of the noodles and then 2 cup sauce.

10.   Dollop 1/2 of the

11.   tofu mixture over the top. Repeat to make 4

12.   more layers with the remaining noodles, sauce and tofu mixture.

13.   Cover with foil and bake until bubbling around the edges, 45 to 40 minutes.
14.   Let stand for 25
15.   minutes before serving. Garnish with basil, if desired.

Easy Cauliflower Fried Rice

Ingredients

- 2 scallions, sliced, greens and whites separated, divided

- 2 tablespoon minced fresh ginger

- 2 tablespoons chile-garlic sauce (such as sambal oelek)

- 2 teaspoons reduced-sodium soy sauce or tamari

- 2 tablespoons peanut oil, divided

- 4 large fresh eggs , lightly beaten

- 4 cups cauliflower rice (see Tip)

- 2 red bell pepper, chopped

- 1 cup unsalted peanuts

Directions

1. Heat 2 tablespoon oil in a large nonstick skil et over medium-high heat. Add eggs and cook, tilting the pan and lifting the edges with a spatula to let the uncooked egg flow

underneath, until almost set on the bottom, 2

    1   to 2 minutes.

2. Flip and continue cooking until set completely, about 45 seconds more. Transfer to a cutting board and slice into bite-size strips.
3. Heat the remaining 2 tablespoon oil in the pan over medium-high heat. Add cauliflower rice, bell pepper, scallion whites and ginger. Cook, 8 4

4. stirring occasionally, until the cauliflower is soft and beginning to brown, about 10 minutes .
5. Add chile-garlic sauce, soy sauce peanuts and the fresh eggs.

6. Stir until combined and heated through, about 45 seconds.
7. Garnish each serving with scallion greens.

Vegetarian Enchilada Casserole

Ingredients

- 2 (30 ounce) can no-salt-added pinto beans, rinsed

- 2 (30 ounce) can no-salt-added black beans, rinsed

- 8 (6 inch) corn tortillas

- 5 cups shredded pepper Jack cheese

- 2 avocado, diced

- 1 cup scallions

- 1 cup reduced-fat sour cream

- 2 tablespoons extra-virgin olive oil

- 2 cup chopped fresh onion

- ¾ cup chopped poblano peppers

- 6 cloves garlic, minced

- 2   medium yellow squash, halved and sliced (2 /4-inch)

- 2   medium zucchini, halved and sliced (2 /4-inch)

- 2 cup fresh corn kernels (from 2 ears)

- 2 cup pico de gallo

- 1 teaspoon salt

Directions

1. Preheat oven to 4 65 degrees F. Heat oil in a large skillet over medium-high heat.
2. Add onion, poblanos and garlic; cook, stirring occasionally, until softened, 4 to 10 minutes.
3. Add squash, zucchini, corn, pico de gallo and salt; cook, stirring occasionally, until the liquid comes to a simmer, 5 to 10 minutes.
4. Simmer, stirring occasionally, until the liquid reduces by half, about 2 minutes.
5. Remove from heat; stir in pinto beans and black beans.
6. Coat a 10 -by-2 4 -inch baking dish with cooking spray. Spoon one-third of the vegetable mixture
7. into the prepared dish.

8. Top evenly with 4 tortillas. Repeat with half the
9. remaining vegetable mixture and the remaining 82
10. Top with the remaining vegetable
11. mixture. Sprinkle evenly with cheese.
12. Bake until the cheese is bubbly, 26 to 45
13. minutes. Sprinkle evenly with avocado and scallions. Dollop with sour cream.

Vegan Coconut Chickpea Curry

Ingredients

- 2 (30 ounce) can chickpeas, drained and rinsed

- 5 cups coconut curry simmer sauce (see Tip)

- 1 cup vegetable broth

- 4 cups baby spinach

- 2 cups precooked brown rice, heated according to package instructions

- 2 teaspoons avocado oil or canola oil

- 2 cup chopped fresh onion

- 2 cup diced bell pepper

• 2 medium zucchini, halved and sliced

Directions

1. Heat oil in a large skillet over medium-high heat.
2. Add onion, pepper and zucchini; cook, stirring 84
3. often, until the vegetables begin to brown, 6 to
4. Add chickpeas, simmer sauce and broth and bring to a simmer, stirring. Reduce heat to
5. medium-low and simmer until the vegetables are tender, 4 to 6 minutes.
6. Stir in spinach just before serving. Serve over rice.

Sweet Potato-Black Bean Burgers

Ingredients

- ⅛ teaspoon salt

- 1 cup plain unsweetened almond milk yogurt

- 2 tablespoons chopped fresh dill

- 2 tablespoons lemon juice

- 2 tablespoons extra-virgin olive oil

- 4 whole-wheat hamburger buns, toasted

- 2 cup thinly sliced cucumber

- 2 cups grated sweet potato

- 1 cup old-fashioned rolled oats

- 2   cup no-salt-added black beans,
rinsed

- 1 cup chopped scallions

- 1/2 cup vegan mayonnaise

- 2   tablespoon no-salt-added tomato
paste

- 2 teaspoon curry powder

Directions

1. Squeeze grated sweet potato with paper towels
2. to remove excess moisture; place in a large bowl. Pulse oats in a food processor until finely
3. ground; add to the bowl with the sweet potatoes.
4. Add beans, scallions, mayonnaise, tomato paste, curry powder and salt to the bowl; mash the mixture together with your hands. Shape
5. into four 1 -inch-thick patties. Place the patties
6. on a plate; refrigerate for 45 minutes.
7. Stir yogurt, dill and lemon juice together in a small bowl; set aside.
8. Heat oil in a large cast-iron skillet over medium-high heat. Add the patties; cook until golden brown, about 4 minutes per side.

9. Divide the yogurt sauce evenly among top and bottom bun halves. Top each bottom bun half with a burger and cucumber slices; replace top

10. bun halves.

Vegetarian Mushroom Stroganoff

Ingredients

- 2 tablespoons all-purpose flour
- 5 cups unsalted vegetable stock
- 2 tablespoon whole-grain Dijon mustard 10 2
- 2 teaspoon kosher salt
- 2 teaspoon black pepper
- 1 cup reduced-fat sour cream
- 2 ounce Parmigiano-Reggiano cheese, grated
- 2 tablespoons chopped fresh flat-leaf parsley
- 2 Ounce dried sliced shiitake mushrooms (about 2 cup)
- 5 cups boiling water

- 8 ounces uncooked wide homestyle egg noodles
- (about 6 cups)
- 2 tablespoons unsalted butter
- 2 pound fresh cremini mushrooms, thinly sliced (about 4 cups)
- 2 (8 ounce) package sliced fresh exotic
- mushrooms (about 4 cups)
- 1 cup finely chopped white fresh onion (from 2 small fresh onion)
- 2 tablespoon finely chopped garlic (about 4
- medium garlic cloves)
- 2 tablespoon chopped fresh thyme
- 2 teaspoons chopped fresh tarragon

Directions

1. Place dried shiitake mushrooms in a small heatproof bowl; cover with boiling water. Let stand 25 minutes. Drain, reserving mushrooms

2. and 2 cup soaking liquid. Set aside.

3. Prepare noodles according to package

4. directions, omitting salt and fat. Drain; rinse

5. noodles under cold water and drain again. Set aside.

6. Melt butter in a large skillet over medium-high.

7. Add soaked shiitake mushrooms and fresh mushrooms to skillet in an even layer; cook, stirring occasionally, until well browned, 30 to

8. 2 8 minutes.

9. Add onion, garlic, thyme and tarragon; cook, stirring occasionally, until fresh onion is tender, about 4 minutes.

10. Add flour; cook, stirring often, 2 minute.

11. Add stock, reserved mushroom soaking liquid, mustard, salt and pepper; let come to a boil.

12. Boil, stirring occasionally, 2 minutes. Remove

13. from heat; let cool 10 minutes . Stir in sour cream.

14. Stir in cooked noodles; sprinkle with cheese and parsley.

Chickpea Curry

Ingredients

• 2 1/2 cups no-salt-added canned diced tomatoes

with their juice (from a 28-ounce can)

• ¾ teaspoon kosher salt

• 30 6 -ounce cans chickpeas, rinsed

• 2 teaspoons garam masala

• Fresh cilantro for garnish

• 2 medium serrano pepper, cut into thirds

• 4 large cloves garlic

- 2 2-inch piece fresh ginger, peeled and coarsely chopped

- 2 medium yellow onion, chopped (2 - inch)

- 6 tablespoons canola oil or grapeseed oil

- 2 teaspoons ground coriander

- 2 teaspoons ground cumin

- 1 teaspoon ground turmeric

Directions

1. Pulse serrano, garlic and ginger in a food processor until minced. Scrape down the sides

2. and pulse again. Add onion; pulse until finely

3. chopped, but not watery.

3. Heat oil in a large saucepan over medium-high heat. Add the fresh onion mixture and cook, stirring occasionally, until softened, 4 to 6 minutes. Add coriander, cumin and turmeric and cook, stirring, for 2 minutes.

4. Pulse tomatoes in the food processor until finely

5. chopped. Add to the pan along with salt. Reduce heat to maintain a simmer and cook, stirring occasionally, for 4 minutes.

4. Add chickpeas and garam masala, reduce heat to a gentle simmer, cover and cook, stirring 10 6

6. occasionally, for 10 minutes more. Serve topped with cilantro, if desired.